THE

ULTIMATE WEIGHT

LOSS PLAN

HOW TO SHED POUNDS, TONE UP, AND

TRANSFORM YOUR BODY FOR LIFE

Elsie M. Weisser

DISCLAIMER

All rights reserved. Do not republish any part of this book publication in any form or by any means, including scanning, photocopying or otherwise, without prior written permission to the copyright holder.

Copyright@2023 By Elsie M. Weisser

Table Of Content

Introduction

Welcome to "The Ultimate Weight Loss Plan: How to Shed Pounds, Tone Up, and Transform Your Body for Life"! If you're reading this, you're likely looking for a way to lose weight, tone up, and improve your overall health and well-being. Losing weight can be a challenging and often frustrating process, but it doesn't have to be. With the right plan, dedication, and support, you can shed pounds, tone up, and transform your body for life. In this guide, we'll provide you with the tools and information you need to achieve your weight loss goals, including tips on healthy eating, exercise, and mindset. We'll also provide you with the support and motivation you need to stay on track and reach your goals. With "The Ultimate Weight Loss Plan", you can take control of your health and create the body and life you've always wanted.

Chapter 1

Introduction To Weight Loss: Setting Your Goals And Understanding The Basics

Welcome to the first chapter of "The Ultimate Weight Loss Plan: How to Shed Pounds, Tone Up, and Transform Your Body for Life"! In this chapter, we'll be focusing on the importance of setting your goals and understanding the basics of weight loss.

Losing weight and improving your health can be a challenging journey, but it's an important and rewarding one. The first step in any weight loss plan is to set your goals. It's important to set specific, achievable goals that are tailored to your individual needs and preferences. This can help you stay motivated and on track with your weight loss efforts.

When setting your goals, it's important to consider the following:

- Why You Want To Lose Weight: Consider your motivations for losing weight and how it will benefit your overall health and well-being.

- How Much Weight You Want To Lose: Set a specific and achievable weight loss goal. It's generally recommended to aim for a weight loss of 1-2 pounds per week.

- How You Will Achieve Your Weight Loss Goals: Consider the changes you will need to make to your diet and exercise routine to achieve your weight loss goals.

- Make Your Goals Measurable: Make sure your goals are measurable, so you can track your progress and stay motivated. For example, instead of setting a goal to "lose weight," set a goal to "lose 10 pounds."

- Set Short-Term And Long-Term Goals: Consider setting both short-term and long-term goals to help you stay motivated and on track. For example, you may set a short-term goal to lose 5 pounds in the next month, and a long-term goal to lose 20 pounds in the next 6 months.

- Remember That Weight Loss Is A Journey: Losing weight and improving your health is a journey, and it's important to be patient and focus on progress, not perfection. Don't get discouraged if you don't see immediate results, and remember to celebrate your small victories along the way.

- Seek Support: Having a support system can be helpful for staying motivated and on track with your weight loss goals. This can include friends and family, a support group, or a healthcare professional.

By following these tips, you can set your weight loss goals and understand the basics of weight loss. Remember to be patient and focus on

progress, and don't be afraid to seek support as

you work towards your goals.

Chapter 2

Nutrition For Weight Loss: Understanding Macronutrients, Counting Calories, And Meal Planning

In this chapter, we'll be focusing on the role of nutrition in weight loss and providing tips and strategies for healthy eating. Proper nutrition is a key component of any successful weight loss plan. What you eat can have a major impact on your weight, as well as your overall health and well-being. Understanding the role of macronutrients, such as protein, carbohydrates, and fat, can help you make informed choices about your diet.

- o Macronutrients: Macronutrients are nutrients that the body needs in large amounts to function properly. There are three main macronutrients: protein, carbohydrates, and fat. Each macronutrient plays a specific role in the body and can have different effects on weight loss.

- o Protein: Protein is essential for building and repairing tissues, and it can also help you feel full and satisfied after meals. Good sources of protein include lean meats, poultry, fish, eggs, dairy products, beans, legumes, nuts, and seeds.

- o Carbohydrates: Carbohydrates provide the body with energy and can be found in a variety of foods, including fruits, vegetables, grains, and legumes. There are two main types of carbohydrates: simple carbs, which are found in sugary foods and drinks, and complex carbs, which are found in whole grains, fruits, and vegetables. It's important to focus on complex carbs, which are higher in fiber and nutrients, rather than simple carbs, which can cause blood sugar spikes and contribute to weight gain.

- o Fat: Fat is a concentrated source of energy and is essential for the absorption of certain vitamins and minerals. There are different types of fat, including saturated, unsaturated, and trans fat. It's important to choose healthy sources of fat, such as avocados, nuts, and olive oil, and limit your intake of unhealthy fats, such as trans fats and saturated fats.

- o Calorie Counting: Counting calories can be helpful when trying to lose weight, as it allows you to track your intake and make sure you're consuming fewer calories than you're burning. To lose weight, you need to create a calorie deficit, which can be achieved by reducing your calorie intake or increasing your calorie expenditure through exercise. However, it's important to remember that not all calories are created equal, and it's important to focus on whole, nutrient-dense foods rather than empty calories from processed or fast foods.

- o Meal Planning: Meal planning involves planning out your meals and snacks in advance. This can help you make sure you're getting the nutrients you need and avoid making unhealthy food choices when you're short on time or feeling hungry. There are many different approaches to meal planning, including prepackaged meal plans, cooking in bulk, and using meal delivery services. By finding a method that works for you, you can create a healthy, sustainable eating plan for weight loss.

With proper understanding of the role of macronutrients, counting calories, and meal planning, you can make informed choices about your diet and create a healthy, sustainable eating plan for weight loss. In the next chapter, we'll delve deeper into the role of exercise in weight loss and provide tips and strategies for getting active.

Chapter 3

Exercise For Weight Loss: Choosing The Right Workouts For Your Body And Goals

In this chapter, we'll be focusing on the role of exercise in weight loss and providing tips and strategies for getting active.

Exercise is an important part of any weight loss plan, as it helps you burn calories and build lean muscle mass. By increasing your muscle mass, you can increase your metabolism and burn more calories even at rest. However, it's important to choose the right workouts for your body and goals.

There are many different types of exercise that can be effective for weight loss, including cardiovascular exercise, strength training, and high-intensity interval training (HIIT).

- Cardiovascular Exercise: Cardiovascular exercise, also known as aerobic exercise, is any activity that gets your heart rate up and improves your cardiovascular health. Examples of cardiovascular exercise include running, cycling, and swimming, dancing, and walking. Cardiovascular exercise can help you burn calories, improve your cardiovascular health, and boost your mood. It's generally recommended to aim for at least 150 minutes of moderate-intensity cardiovascular exercise per week, or 75 minutes of vigorous-intensity exercise.

- Strength Training: Strength training, also known as resistance training, involves using weights, resistance bands, or your own body weight to work against resistance and build lean muscle mass. Strength training can help you increase your metabolism, improve your bone density, and improve your overall strength and fitness. It's generally recommended to aim for at least two strength training sessions per week, working all major muscle groups.

- High-Intensity Interval Training (HIIT): High-intensity interval training (HIIT) is a type of exercise that involves short bursts of high-intensity exercise followed by periods of rest. HIIT can be very effective for weight loss as it can help you burn a lot of calories in a short amount of time. It can also improve your cardiovascular health, boost your metabolism, and increase your fitness level. HIIT can be done with a variety of exercises, such as running, cycling, or bodyweight exercises, and can be customized to fit your fitness level.

It's important to remember that everybody is different and it's important to find an exercise routine that works for you and fits into your lifestyle. It's generally recommended to aim for at least 150 minutes of moderate-intensity exercise per week, or a combination of moderate- and vigorous-intensity exercise, and to include strength training at least twice per week. By finding an exercise routine that you enjoy and that fits into your lifestyle, you can make exercise a sustainable part of your weight loss journey.

By choosing the right workouts for your body and goals, you can make exercise a key part of your weight loss plan and improve your overall health and well-being. In the next chapter, we'll delve deeper into the importance of lifestyle changes for weight loss and provide tips and strategies for incorporating healthy habits into your daily routine.

Chapter 4

Making Lifestyle Changes For Weight Loss: Incorporating Healthy Habits Into Your Daily Routine

Losing weight and improving your health is not just about diet and exercise, it's also about making lifestyle changes that support your weight loss goals. This includes things like getting enough sleep, managing stress, and staying hydrated.

Here are a few tips for incorporating healthy habits into your daily routine:

❖ Getting Enough Sleep: Getting enough sleep is essential for weight loss and overall health. During sleep, the body repairs and regenerates tissues, and it's also when the body releases growth hormone, which helps to build muscle mass. Poor sleep can disrupt hormone production and contribute to weight gain. Aim for 7-9 hours of sleep per night to support your weight loss goals and overall health.

❖ Managing Stress: Chronic stress can contribute to weight gain by increasing the production of the hormone cortisol, which can lead to abdominal fat storage. It's important to find ways to manage stress, such as through relaxation techniques, exercise, or talking to a therapist.

❖ Staying Hydrated: Drinking enough water is essential for overall health, and it can also help you feel full and satisfied, which can be helpful when trying to lose weight. Aim for at least 8 cups of water per day, and more if you're physically active or it's hot outside.

❖ Planning Ahead: Meal planning and packing healthy snacks can help you stay on track and avoid making unhealthy food choices when you're short on time. By planning out your meals and snacks in advance, you can make sure you're getting the nutrients you need and avoid getting caught without a healthy option.

❖ Finding Support: Surrounding yourself with supportive friends and family, or joining a support group, can help you stay motivated and accountable on your weight loss journey. Having a support system can help you overcome obstacles and setbacks and stay on track with your goals.

By incorporating these healthy habits into your daily routine, you can create a sustainable, healthy lifestyle that supports your weight loss goals. It's important to remember that everyone is different, and it's important to find what works for you and your lifestyle.

Chapter 5

Overcoming Obstacles And Setbacks: How To Stay Motivated And On Track

Losing weight and improving your health is not always a smooth, straight path. There will be obstacles and setbacks along the way, and it's important to have strategies in place to help you stay motivated and on track. Here are a few tips for overcoming obstacles and setbacks:

> ➢ Don't be too hard on yourself: It's normal to have ups and downs, and it's important to remember that progress is not always a straight line. Be kind to yourself and don't beat yourself up over setbacks or mistakes. Instead, focus on the progress you've made

and the positive changes you've implemented.

➢ Keep things in perspective: Remembering why you started on your weight loss journey and what your long-term goals are can help you stay motivated and keep things in perspective when you face setbacks. It can be helpful to write down your goals and refer back to them when you're feeling discouraged.

➢ Focus on progress, not perfection: It's important to celebrate small victories and focus on the progress you've made, rather than striving for perfection. Recognize and appreciate the progress you've made, and don't let setbacks discourage you.

➢ Find ways to stay motivated: There are many ways to stay motivated on your weight loss journey. Surrounding yourself with supportive friends and family, joining a support group, or finding an accountability partner can all be helpful. You can also try setting rewards for yourself or finding new, enjoyable ways to stay active.

➢ Don't give up: It's normal to have ups and downs, but it's important to keep going and not give up on your weight loss goals. Remember that progress takes time, and it's important to be patient and consistent. If you're feeling stuck or unsure of what to do, consider seeking the help of a healthcare professional or a licensed mental health therapist.

By following these tips, you can stay motivated and on track on your weight loss journey, even when faced with obstacles and setbacks. Remember that progress is not always a straight line, and it's important to be patient and consistent, and to focus on the progress you've made.

Chapter 6

The Importance Of Self-Care And Stress Management For Weight Loss

Self-care and stress management are important components of any weight loss plan, as they can help you feel more balanced and energized and support your overall health and well-being. Here are a few tips for incorporating self-care and stress management into your weight loss journey:

- ✓ Making time for yourself: It's important to set aside time for activities that nourish and recharge you, whether it's reading a book, taking a bath, or going for a walk. This can help you feel more balanced and energized and better able to handle the demands of daily life.

✓ Practicing relaxation techniques: Relaxation techniques such as meditation, deep breathing, or yoga can help you manage stress and feel more calm and centered. These techniques can also help you sleep better and improve your overall well-being.

✓ Getting enough sleep: Aiming for 7-9 hours of sleep per night can support your weight loss goals and overall health. Poor sleep can disrupt hormone production and contribute to weight gain.

✓ Taking breaks: It's important to take breaks from work and other demands to give yourself time to rest and recharge. This can help you feel more energized and better able to handle the demands of daily life.

✓ Seeking support: If you're feeling overwhelmed or stressed, it can be helpful to seek the support of a healthcare professional or a licensed mental health therapist. These professionals can provide guidance and support to help you manage stress and improve your overall well-being.

By incorporating self-care and stress management into your weight loss journey, you can feel more balanced and energized and support your overall health and well-being. It's important to remember that everyone is different and it's important to find what works for you and your lifestyle.

Chapter 7

Incorporating Strength Training Into Your Weight Loss Plan

In this chapter, we'll be focusing on the importance of strength training for weight loss and providing tips for incorporating it into your weight loss plan.

Strength training, also known as resistance training, involves using weights, resistance bands, or your own body weight to work against resistance and build lean muscle mass. In addition to improving your strength and fitness, strength training has several benefits for weight loss, including:

- Increasing your metabolism: Building lean muscle mass can increase your metabolism, which means you'll burn more calories even at rest.

- Burning calories: Strength training can help you burn calories and contribute to a calorie deficit, which is necessary for weight loss.

- Improving body composition: Strength training can help you lose fat and build lean muscle mass, which can improve your body composition and help you look and feel your best.

It's generally recommended to aim for at least two strength training sessions per week, working all major muscle groups. It's also important to vary your workouts and use a variety of exercises and resistance levels to challenge your muscles and prevent plateaus.

There are many different ways to incorporate strength training into your weight loss plan, including lifting weights at the gym, using resistance bands at home, or trying bodyweight exercises like push-ups, squats, and lunges. You can also try taking a strength training class or working with a personal trainer to learn proper form and technique and to create a personalized strength training plan.

It's important to start slowly and gradually increase the intensity and difficulty of your workouts as you become stronger. It's also important to listen to your body and rest as needed. Strength training should not be painful, and it's important to stop if you experience any discomfort or pain.

Incorporating strength training into your weight loss plan can help you increase your metabolism, burn calories, and improve your body composition. It's an important component of any weight loss plan and can help you look and feel your best. In the next chapter, we'll delve into the importance of cardiovascular exercise for weight loss and provide tips for getting active.

Chapter 8

High-Intensity Interval Training For Weight Loss

High-intensity interval training (HIIT) is a type of exercise that involves short bursts of high-intensity exercise followed by periods of rest. HIIT can be very effective for weight loss as it can help you burn a lot of calories in a short amount of time. It can also improve your cardiovascular health, boost your metabolism, and increase your fitness level.

HIIT can be done with a variety of exercises, such as running, cycling, or bodyweight exercises, and can be customized to fit your fitness level. A typical HIIT workout might involve repeating a circuit of exercises for a set number of rounds, with each exercise performed at high intensity for a specific amount of time followed by a rest period.

It's important to start slowly with HIIT and gradually increase the intensity and duration of your workouts as you become more fit. It's also important to listen to your body and stop if you experience any discomfort or pain.

I.   Benefits of HIIT: In addition to helping you burn a lot of calories in a short amount of time, HIIT has several other benefits for weight loss and overall health. HIIT can improve your cardiovascular health, boost your metabolism, and increase your fitness level. It can also be a time-efficient way to exercise, as HIIT workouts can be done in as little as 20-30 minutes.

II. Types of HIIT exercises: HIIT can be done with a variety of exercises, such as running, cycling, or bodyweight exercises like squats, lunges, and push-ups. You can also use equipment such as a treadmill, stationary bike, or jump rope for your HIIT workouts. The key is to perform the exercises at high intensity for a specific amount of time followed by a rest period.

III. Customizing HIIT for your fitness level: HIIT can be customized to fit your fitness level by adjusting the intensity and duration of the high-intensity intervals and rest periods. For example, if you're just starting out, you might start with shorter intervals and longer rest periods, and gradually increase the intensity and decrease the rest periods as you become more fit. It's important to start slowly and gradually increase the intensity and duration of your workouts as you become more fit.

IV.   Warming up and cooling down: It's important to warm up before starting a HIIT workout to get your muscles ready for the high-intensity intervals. This can involve a few minutes of light cardio and some dynamic stretches.

Incorporating HIIT into your fitness routine can be a great way to boost your weight loss efforts and improve your overall fitness. It's important to

remember to warm up before starting a HIIT

workout

Chapter 9

The Role Of Cardiovascular Exercise In Weight Loss

Cardiovascular exercise, also known as aerobic exercise, involves sustained, rhythmic movement of the large muscle groups and is designed to increase your heart rate and improve your cardiovascular health. Cardiovascular exercise can be an effective tool for weight loss as it can help you burn calories, boost your metabolism, and improve your overall fitness.

There are many different types of cardiovascular exercise, including walking, running, cycling, swimming, and dancing. It's generally recommended to aim for at least 150 minutes of moderate-intensity cardiovascular exercise per week, or 75 minutes of vigorous-intensity exercise, as recommended by the Centers for Disease Control and Prevention (CDC).

Incorporating cardiovascular exercise into your weight loss plan can help you burn calories, boost your metabolism, and improve your overall fitness. It's important to choose activities that you enjoy and that fit your fitness level, and to start slowly and gradually increase the intensity and duration of your workouts as you become more fit. It's also important to listen to your body and stop if you experience any discomfort or pain.

In the next chapter, we'll delve into the role of flexibility and stretching in weight loss and provide tips for incorporating stretching into your fitness routine.

Chapter 10

The Benefits Of Yoga And Mindfulness For Weight Loss"

Welcome to the tenth chapter of "The Ultimate Weight Loss Plan: How to Shed Pounds, Tone Up, and Transform Your Body for Life"! In this chapter, we'll be focusing on the benefits of yoga and mindfulness for weight loss and providing tips for incorporating these practices into your fitness routine.

Yoga and mindfulness are practices that involve physical postures, breathing techniques, and meditation or mindfulness techniques, and can be an effective part of a weight loss plan. Yoga can help improve flexibility, strength, and balance, and it has also been shown to reduce stress and improve overall well-being.

Incorporating yoga and mindfulness into your weight loss plan can help you in several ways:

1. Reducing stress: Yoga and mindfulness practices can help reduce stress and improve overall well-being, which can be helpful when trying to lose weight.

2. Improving flexibility and strength: Yoga can help improve flexibility, strength, and balance, which can be beneficial for overall health and fitness.

3. Reducing emotional eating: Practicing mindfulness can help you become more aware of your eating habits and identify any emotional triggers that may lead to unhealthy eating habits.

4. Finding a class or practice that fits your fitness level: It's important to choose a class or practice that fits your fitness level to ensure that you can participate safely and comfortably. If you're new to yoga, it can be helpful to start with a beginner's class or practice. If you have any injuries or medical conditions, it's important to consult with a healthcare professional before starting a yoga or mindfulness practice.

5. Listening to your body: It's important to listen to your body and stop if you experience any discomfort or pain during a yoga or mindfulness practice. If you have any injuries or medical conditions, it's important to modify poses or practices as needed and to consult with a healthcare professional before starting a yoga or mindfulness practice.

6. Being consistent in your practice: To see the full benefits of yoga and mindfulness, it's important to be consistent in your practice. This can mean setting aside time for a daily practice or attending a weekly class.

Consistency can help you build a strong foundation and see progress in your practice over time.

49

Incorporating yoga and mindfulness into your weight loss plan can be a powerful tool for reducing stress, improving flexibility and strength, and reducing emotional eating. It's important to find a practice that works for you and to be consistent in your practice to see the full benefits.

Chapter 11

The Role Of Sleep In Weight Loss

Sleep is an important part of any weight loss plan, as it can impact your energy levels, appetite, and overall health and well-being. Getting enough quality sleep can help you feel more rested and energized, which can make it easier to stick to your weight loss goals.

Here are a few tips for getting a good night's sleep:

✓ Set a consistent sleep schedule: Going to bed and waking up at the same time every day can help regulate your body's natural sleep-wake cycle and improve the quality of your sleep.

✓ Create a relaxing bedtime routine: Establishing a relaxing bedtime routine can help you wind down and prepare for sleep. This can include activities such as reading, meditating, or taking a warm bath.

✓ Make your sleep environment comfortable: Creating a comfortable sleep environment can help you get a good night's sleep. This can include a comfortable bed, a cool, dark, and quiet room, and a comfortable sleep temperature.

✓ Avoid screens before bed: The blue light emitted by screens can disrupt your body's natural sleep-wake cycle, so it's best to avoid screens for at least an hour before bed.

By following these tips, you can improve the quality of your sleep and support your weight loss efforts. In the next chapter, we'll delve into the role of hydration in weight loss and provide tips for staying hydrated.

Chapter 12

How To Track Your Progress And Stay Accountable

Tracking your progress can be a powerful tool for staying motivated and on track with your weight loss goals. It can also help you identify any areas that may need improvement and make adjustments to your plan as needed.

There are several ways to track your progress, including:

➢ Weighing yourself : Weighing yourself regularly can provide valuable information about your weight loss progress. It's important to remember that weight can fluctuate due to factors such as water intake and hormone levels, so it's best to weigh yourself at the same time each day and look for trends over time rather than focusing on any one individual weigh-in.

- ➢ Measuring your waist circumference: Measuring your waist circumference can provide information about your body composition and can be an indicator of abdominal fat, which is associated with an increased risk of chronic disease.

- ➢ Taking progress photos: Taking progress photos can help you see the changes in your body over time and can be a powerful motivator.

- ➢ Keeping a food and exercise journal: Keeping a journal of what you eat and your physical activity can help you identify patterns and make adjustments to your eating and exercise habits as needed.

By tracking your progress and staying accountable, you can stay motivated and on track with your weight loss goals. In the next chapter, we'll delve into the importance of finding a support system for weight loss and provide tips for building a supportive network.

Chapter 13

Making Weight Loss A Sustainable, Long-Term Lifestyle Change

Losing weight and keeping it off can be a challenge, but it's important to remember that weight loss is not a short-term fix. To successfully lose weight and keep it off, it's important to make healthy habits a part of your daily routine.

Here are a few tips for making weight loss a sustainable, long-term lifestyle change:

❖ Focus on healthy habits, not just weight loss: Instead of focusing solely on weight loss, focus on incorporating healthy habits into your daily routine. This can include eating a balanced diet, getting regular physical activity, getting enough sleep, and managing stress.

❖ Make gradual changes: Instead of trying to overhaul your entire lifestyle at once, focus on making gradual changes. This can make it easier to stick to your healthy habits and create lasting change.

❖ Find balance: It's important to find a balance between healthy habits and flexibility. Don't feel like you have to be perfect all the time, as this can be unrealistic and unsustainable. Instead, focus on making healthy choices most of the time and allowing yourself some flexibility.

❖ Seek support: Finding a support system can be a valuable tool for helping you stay motivated and on track with your healthy habits. This can include friends and family, a support group, or a healthcare professional.

❖ Identify and address any barriers to healthy habits: Identify any barriers that may be preventing you from adopting healthy habits, such as lack of time or access to healthy food options. By addressing these barriers, you can make it easier to stick to your healthy habits.

❖ Find activities that you enjoy: It's important to find physical activities that you enjoy, as this can make it more likely that you'll stick to an exercise routine. This can be anything from walking or running to dancing or yoga.

❖ Don't get too caught up in the scale: While tracking your weight can be a useful tool, it's important to remember that weight loss is not the only indicator of progress. Focus on other markers of progress, such as improved fitness, better sleep, and increased energy levels.

❖ Remember that progress takes time: Weight loss is a journey, and it's important to be patient and remember that progress takes time. Don't get discouraged if you don't see immediate results, and remember to celebrate your small victories along the way.

By following these tips, you can make weight loss a sustainable, long-term lifestyle change and create lasting healthy habits. It's important to be patient and focus on the journey, as well as the destination, and to celebrate your progress and accomplishments along the way.

Chapter 14

How To Maintain Your Weight Loss And Continue Improving Your Health

Congratulations on reaching your weight loss goals! Losing weight is a significant accomplishment, and it's important to celebrate your success. However, it's also important to remember that weight loss is a journey, and maintaining your weight loss and continuing to improve your health is an ongoing process.

Here are a few tips for maintaining your weight loss and continuing to improve your health:

- Continue to follow a healthy diet: To maintain your weight loss, it's important to continue to follow a healthy diet that is rich in whole foods, such as fruits, vegetables, whole grains, and lean proteins.

- Stay Active: Regular physical activity is important for both weight maintenance and overall health. Aim to get at least 150 minutes of moderate-intensity exercise or 75 minutes of vigorous-intensity exercise per week, as recommended by the Centers for Disease Control and Prevention (CDC).

- Monitor Your Weight: While it's important not to get too caught up in the scale, it can be helpful to periodically weigh yourself to monitor your weight and make any necessary adjustments to your diet and exercise routine.

- Seek support: Having a support system can be helpful for maintaining your weight loss and continuing to improve your health. This can include friends and family, a support group, or a healthcare professional.

- Practice stress management: Chronic stress can impact your weight and overall health, so it's important to find healthy ways to manage stress. This can include activities such as exercise, meditation, or spending time with loved ones.

- Get enough sleep: Getting enough sleep is important for both weight maintenance and overall health. Aim for 7-9 hours of sleep per night.

- Stay hydrated: Drinking enough water is important for weight maintenance and overall health. Aim for 8-8 ounces of water per day.

- Don't be too hard on yourself: It's important to be kind to yourself and remember that it's okay to have setbacks or make mistakes. It's important to focus on progress, not perfection, and to celebrate your small victories along the way.

By following these tips, you can successfully maintain your weight loss and continue to improve your health. It's important to find what works for you and to be consistent in your healthy habits to see the full benefits. Congratulations on your weight loss journey and all that you have

accomplished!

Chapter 15

Wrapping It Up: Celebrating Your Achievements And Setting New Goals

Congratulations on completing "The Ultimate Weight Loss Plan: How to Shed Pounds, Tone Up, and Transform Your Body for Life"! Losing weight and improving your health is a significant accomplishment, and it's important to celebrate your achievements.

Here are a few tips for celebrating your achievements and setting new goals:

- o Take some time to reflect on your journey: Take a few moments to reflect on your weight loss journey and all that you have accomplished. Think about what you have learned and the challenges you have overcome.

- o Celebrate your accomplishments: Take some time to celebrate your accomplishments, whether it's treating yourself to something special or sharing your success with loved ones.

- o Set new goals: Now that you have reached your weight loss goals, it's important to set new goals to continue improving your health and well-being. This can be anything from maintaining your weight loss to improving your fitness level or trying a new activity.

- o Reflect on your progress: Take some time to reflect on the progress you have made and the healthy habits you have developed. This can help you feel more confident and motivated to continue on your journey.

- o Share your success: Sharing your success with others can be a powerful motivator and can help you stay accountable. Consider sharing your story with friends and family, or joining a support group or online community to connect with others who are also working on improving their health.

- o Reward yourself: Treat yourself to something special as a reward for your hard work and dedication. This can be anything from a new outfit to a relaxing massage or a fun activity that you enjoy.

o   Set realistic goals: It's important to set goals that are realistic and achievable, as this can help you stay motivated and on track. Consider setting both short-term and long-term goals, and remember to be patient and focus on progress, not perfection.

By following these tips, you can celebrate your achievements and set new goals to continue improving your health and well-being. Remember to be kind to yourself, focus on progress, and celebrate your small victories along the way. Congratulations on your weight loss journey and all that you have accomplished!